Back Care

Second Edition

Second Edition Editor:

Augustus A. White III, M.D., Dr.Med.Sci.
Professor of Orthopaedic Surgery, Harvard Medical School
Former Orthopaedic Surgeon-in-Chief,
Beth Israel Hospital, Boston

First Edition Author:

Arthur E. Grant, M.D., Professor Emeritus and former chairman, Department of Physical Medicine and Rehabilitation, The University of Texas Medical School at San Antonio

Second Edition Consultant:

Ib R. Odderson, M.D., Ph.D., Assistant Professor, Department of Rehabilitation Medicine, University of Washington Medical Center, Seattle; Medical Director, Rehabilitation Services, Overlake Hospital Medical Center, Bellevue; and Chief Rehabilitation Consultant, Lake Vue Gardens Convalescent Center, Kirkland, Washington

Publisher's General Editor: **Murray A. Swanson**

Medic Publishing Co.
P.O. Box 238, Preston, WA 98050
Voice 425-222-0844 FAX 425-222-0845

Contents

Perhaps your back problem requires special medical treatment. Even if it does not, you need medical supervision. Only a physician is prepared to evaluate and treat your total condition. If there is conflict between what he or she says and what is written here, disregard what is written and follow your physician's advice. Also keep in mind that each person responds a little differently. The advice given, although correct for most people, *may not be correct for you.* Pay close attention to the warnings and be sensitive to your body's response.

Introduction

Most backaches can be treated simply and effectively. That's because *common problems involve soft tissues (muscles, ligaments),* which may be weak, tight, irritated, or damaged. The program in this booklet is designed to help heal these tissues and to protect them from further problems.

This program also helps greatly when there is an *underlying problem with other structures.* The discs (pads) between vertebrae deteriorate. They may bulge and sometimes rupture (herniate). The facet joints, which connect the back parts of the vertebrae, become irritated. These and other changes can cause pain. This program stimulates circulation, improves alignment, strengthens the surrounding muscles, and reduces stress to these areas.

Introduction, continued

The crucial part of the lower back is the area of the five lumbar vertebrae. Here all forward and backward bending of the back occurs. The lumbar spine curves forward, and the vertebrae must be supported the way a leaning tree is supported by stakes and wires. *Back muscles* provide this support. And because the vertebrae are stacked on the pelvis, pelvic position also affects low back position. *Muscles of the hips and abdomen* control pelvic position.

If the upper part of the pelvis moves forward and downward from its normal position, the forward curve (lordosis) in the lumbar area increases. The spine moves forward toward the abdomen and the result may be *swayback,* too much lumbar lordosis.

The *abdominal muscles* attach to the upper part of the pelvis. Weakness of these muscles is a major cause of swayback. The *gluteal muscles* in the buttocks attach to the back of the lower pelvis, so weakness of these muscles also causes forward rotation. With swayback, the muscles, ligaments, and other tissues of the back may become short and tight.

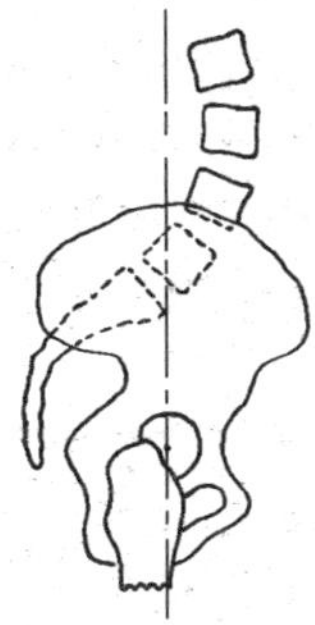

Top of pelvis forward causes swayback

Posture is the position of your body both at rest and during activities. Swayback is a form of poor posture. In good posture, the pelvis is tilted back to its normal position. This booklet shows habits and simple exercises to make good posture of the pelvis and low back your natural position. Returning the low back to its normal slight curve may reduce pain and, if maintained, make future attacks of back pain less likely.

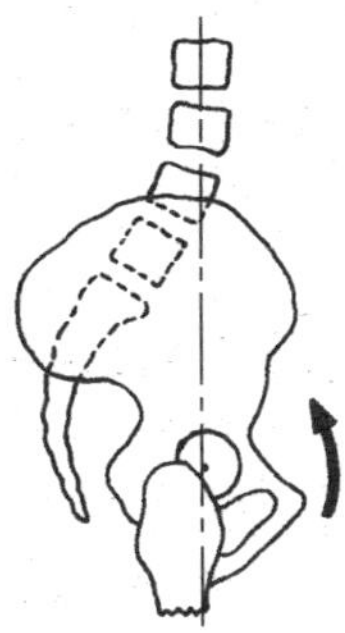

Top of pelvis tilted backward corrects swayback

Possible Underlying Problems

A portion of the lumbar spine is shown without muscles and ligaments.

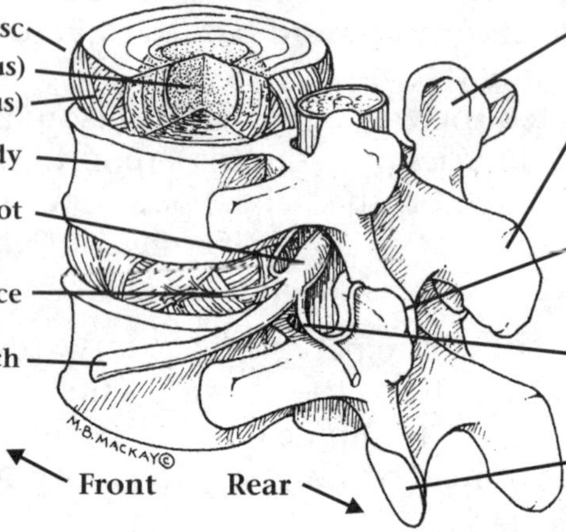

The disc is like a cushion between the vertebrae. It has a soft gelatin-like center and a thick, tough outer wall. The discs are firmly attached, top and bottom, and cannot "slip." They begin to dry out at an early age and gradually lose height and resilience. This drying of the disc is the most basic underlying problem. One of the benefits of exercise and other recommendations in this booklet is likely to be healthier discs.

The disc wall may bulge and even tear. The soft material from the nucleus may pass through the damaged wall. The bulge or soft material may press on a nerve root, causing sharp leg pain—*sciatica*. This happens in only a few percent of cases. Your doctor will probably be able to tell if you have this condition. It will usually heal if you allow it time, aided by this program.

Facet joints can become irritated. Reduced height in the disc can put greater forces on these joints, causing wear. Wear in a joint is called osteoarthritis. Exercise and good posture in all your activities help protect against pain starting in the facet joints.

Nerve roots leaving the spinal canal travel through a narrow passageway between two vertebrae. As a person ages, this area tends to get smaller because of the loss of disc height and the growth of bone spurs (osteophytes). The narrowing, called *spinal stenosis,* may irritate nerve roots. Typically this kind of nerve irritation causes dull pain and/or numbness in the legs. Although walking often brings on the pain, certain exercises are helpful.

FIRST AID

How to speed recovery from a painful back attack

See Your Doctor

Unusual problems need to be checked out by your doctor. Call *right away* if you have numbness in the genital or rectal area, major leg weakness, or lack of bladder or bowel control.

Bed Rest

Bed rest, at once or as soon as practical, can be very helpful. Get up as little as possible, but limit this kind of rest to two or three days. In some cases, as with leg pain, your doctor may order more, but prolonged bed rest weakens the body and has other ill effects. Find the resting position most comfortable for you. Usually this is on your back with knees up and supported by a blanket roll or heavy pillows. Another position is on your side with knees bent and a pillow between them.

Ice and Heat

Ice packs are usually better in the first forty-eight hours. To avoid frostbite, limit ice to 15 or 20 minutes every hour and use a towel over the pack. Some people like an "ice massage," ice cubes moved about directly on the skin. After the second day, use heat. Some people like "moist heat" heating pads (be careful not to burn yourself). A hot water bottle or microwave gel pack is preferred by those who want to avoid the electromagnetic radiation from a heating pad. Avoid *continuous* heat or ice.

A Position of Relief

If you get your back into a relaxed position and stay there for awhile, you may get quick relief. The "Z" position often helps.

Lie on floor with your lower legs and feet on a low table, hassock, or low chair. Use a pillow or pad for height or comfort. Thighs should be nearly vertical. Put a thin cushion or towel under buttocks (not under back). Put a small pillow under your head.

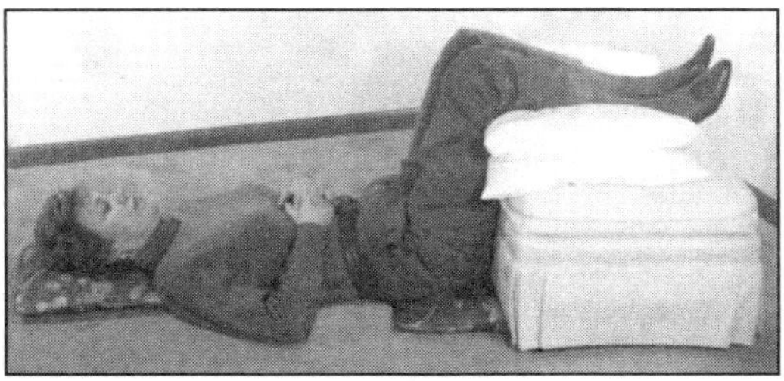

The "Z" Position

More Positions of Relief

It takes trial and error to find the positions that relieve pain. Stop any that make your back hurt more. The clues in the boxes will help.

Extension Positions

If back pain is worse when you *sit* or *bend forward,* these positions are likely to help. They move you "away from pain."

Standing Extension. While standing with feet apart and hands on buttocks, push hips forward and gently bend backward while looking up. Hold several seconds. Keep knees straight. Relax, repeat. Do several times a day, especially after sitting.

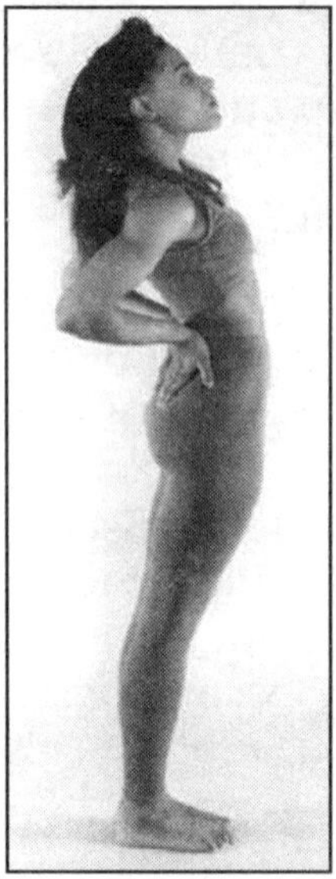

Standing Extension

Prone. First try lying on your stomach without any raising. If this hurts, put a small pillow under the top of your pelvis. As pain lessens, remove pillow. When able, advance to:

Prone on Forearms. Rest on forearms like a child watching TV. Try 3 to 5 minutes. A pillow may be used instead of forearms.

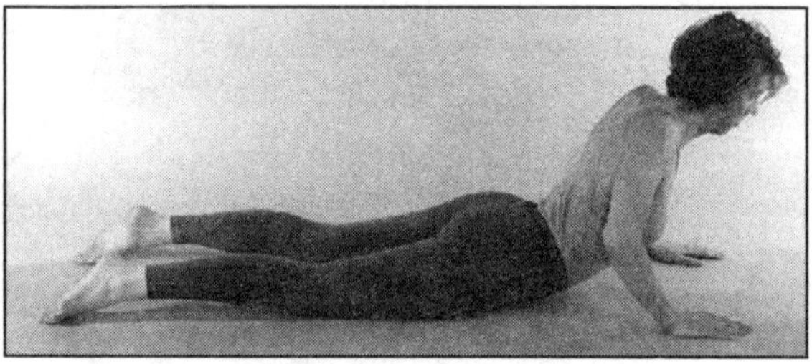

Press-up

Press-up. Advance to this when you can. Lie on your stomach. Place your hands palms down on the floor near your shoulders. Slowly push your upper body up. Let your hips sag. Keep chin in. Stop raising when you feel tension. Elbows need not be straight at first, but later you will probably be able to lock them. Hold for several seconds (breathe naturally), then return to floor. Relax and repeat. Start with 3 repetitions. Work up to 10.

If you have pain *mainly* in a leg rather than in the back, extension positions (above) are likely to help. So might the "Z" position, pg. 5. See also page 18.

Flexion Positions

If back pain is worse when you *bend backward,* these positions are likely to help. They move you "away from the pain."

Standing Pelvic Tilt. Stand with back against a wall with feet about 12 inches from the wall. Squeeze your buttocks together as if gripping a coin. Pull in your abdomen. The space behind your back should be gone. Hold several seconds. Relax and repeat a few times. With practice, you will be able to bring your feet closer to the wall and still have a flat back. Do this several times a day. A wall is helpful at first but not necessary later.

Lying Pelvic Tilt. Lie on back on floor, knees bent. Squeeze buttocks, pull in abdomen. Low back goes flat. Hold several seconds. Relax, repeat. Work up to 10 times.

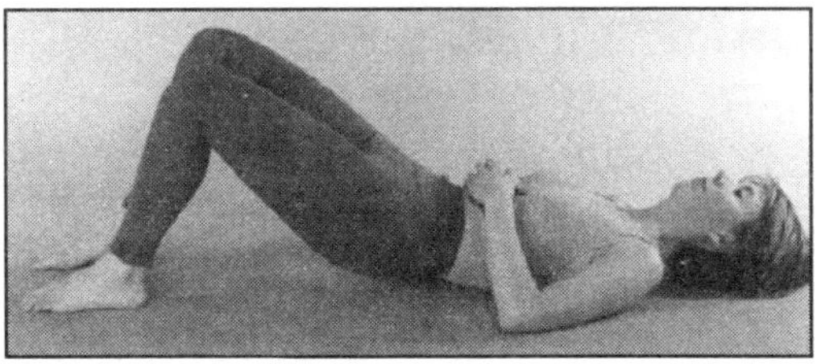

Advanced Pelvic Tilt. Same as Lying Pelvic Tilt, except also raise buttocks slightly—an inch or so. Do not push with feet.

Sitting Bend. Sit in a chair, flatten back (do pelvic tilt), knees apart. Bend *slowly* at waist, hands reaching toward ankles, head ending near knees. Hold briefly, sit up, relax and repeat. *Do not force* for extra distance as this will cause pressure inside discs.

Double Knee to Chest. Lie on back on floor, knees bent. Do the pelvic tilt. Hold low back on floor as you begin. With hand over knee (or under), gently pull one knee toward chest. Hold it while pulling other knee toward chest. Hold both for 10 seconds. Return one knee at a time, relax, and repeat. Do not straighten knee when returning. Work up to 10 repetitions.

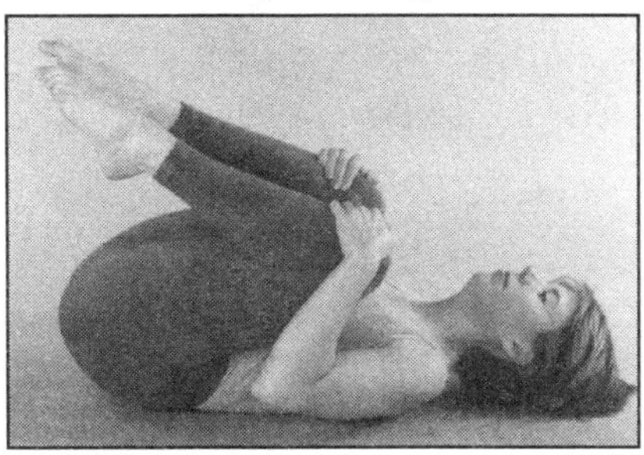

Leg pain that is *dull* and worse if *walking* suggests *stenosis.* See page 4, last paragraph. Try above flexion positions.

RELIEF IN DAILY ACTIVITIES

How to protect your back at all times

The next few pages are about your position in all your activities. A little change in your habits together with certain simple exercises will do wonders for your back.

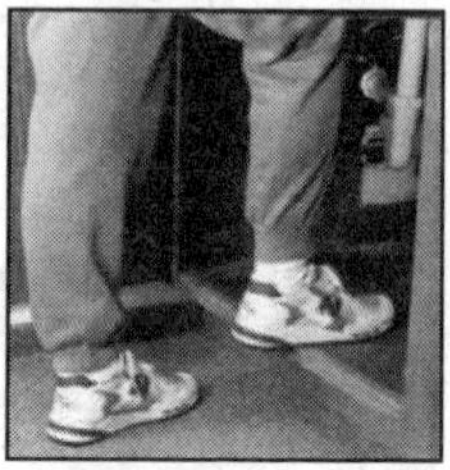

Kitchen sinks have hidden foot rests.

Standing. Stand tall. Slouching shoulders forward is bad for the back. Practice keeping your *shoulders slightly back* and your chin a little tucked in.

Pelvic tilt while standing. When you must stand for a long period, occasionally *tilt your pelvis* as described on page 7.

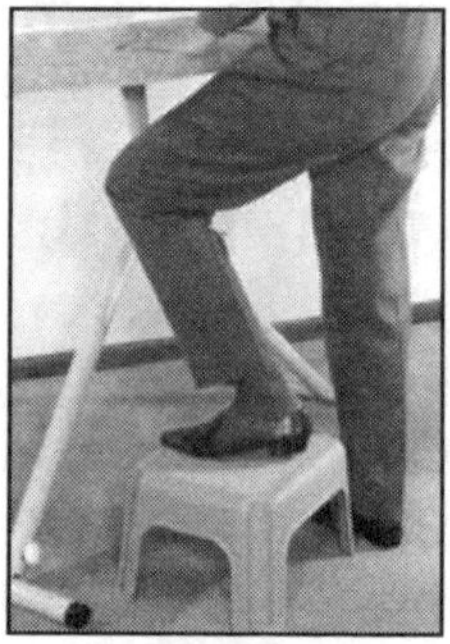

Keep a stool handy for standing tasks.

Foot up. One foot on a stool or rail improves back posture—helpful for bank tellers, surgeons, and others who stand a lot. Also useful for home tasks—washing dishes, ironing.

Changing position. Don't stay in one position very long. Relax shoulders, then dangle arms occasionally.

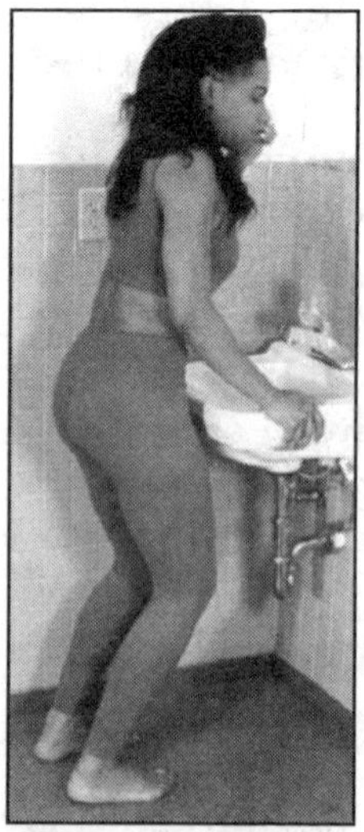

Bend knees more. Bend back less.

Leaning. Whenever possible, avoid leaning from the waist. When you must reach down, *bend your knees* and use the lifting principles (page 11). Two of the exercises in the conditioning group (page 21) strengthen muscles for this purpose.

High heels. Low-heeled shoes are usually recommended because many people get relief from switching to lower heels. But there are exceptions—some people do better with higher heels. Men can try higher heeled boots.

Sleeping

A mattress must support your body in two ways. (1) It must be *firm enough to keep your spine horizontal.* Your body must not sag as if in a hammock. (2) It must *follow your curves.* This is called good *conformity.* Test for conformity by lying on your side—the mattress should come up strongly into the waist area. To meet the first requirement, modern mattresses have firm springs, and some have extra support in the middle area. To meet the second, a large number of smaller springs is helpful.

Your weight and your shape affect your choice of mattress. A heavy person needs heavy springs—more firmness. Others need less firmness so that hips will sink in a little. If your hips are much wider than your waist, you will need lots of conformity so that waist and lumbar spine are supported. Be sure to try out mattresses in the showroom before you buy. Take your time.

A modern **foundation** gives a strong, flat support to the mattress. When the foundation sags and you can't afford a new one, a **bed board** should help. Use 3/4 inch plywood between the mattress and the foundation. A piece 4 feet wide by 5 feet long (easily cut at a lumber yard) is usually large enough for a double or queen size bed. A king size bed (76 inches wide) requires two 3 feet by 5 feet pieces. Bear in mind that a bed board will not fix a poor mattress.

Waterbeds, some people say, are helpful for their backs; others say their backs are worse. Newer models have extra support in the lumbar area. Try one at least overnight before you buy.

Sleeping position. *On your side is best.* Put arms in front and partially curl your body. A pillow should fit the space between mattress and head. Head should stay in line with body, tilted neither up nor down. Foam pillows tend to hold head too high.

Sleeping on your back is okay if your knees are raised and supported. A blanket roll or large pillows can be used temporarily, but adjustable beds (either rented or purchased) are easier. For your head, use no pillow or a very thin one.

Sleeping on your stomach strains the back. If that is your only comfortable position, try a thin pillow under your pelvis.

Sitting

Basic rules. If you sit for long periods, (1) take a proper position, (2) use a chair with good support, (3) get up and move about occasionally, (4) exercise regularly.

Proper position. Sit with low back supported by the back of the chair. Do not lean forward except briefly. Knees should be a little higher than the hips, and thighs should be well supported. Feet should be firmly on floor or (if necessary for a short person) on a low stool or phone book. The ideal chair firmly supports the lumbar area but *not* with a narrow band. The back rest should rise at least to the top of the lumbar area and preferably to shoulders. Seat should adjust for height and be deep enough to support the thighs. Tilting action (both seat and back moving together) is good for frequent relief from one position. Arm rests also help.

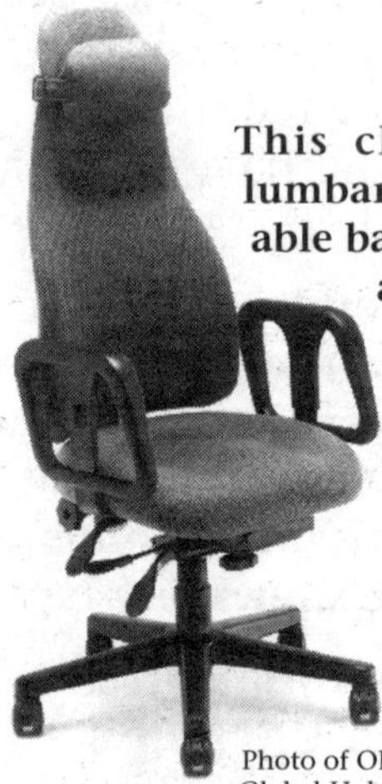

This chair has strong lumbar support, adjustable backrest, adjustable armrests, and ample thigh support. Both seat and back can be tilted and locked backward to reduce force on the spine.

Photo of OBUS Forme™ chair courtesy Global Upholstery Co., Toronto

Driving a car or truck. Sit back. Don't lean forward. Adjust seat so pedals are reached easily. Knees should be slightly higher than hips. Add a back support if seat back does not firmly support lumbar area (see below). On trips, stop frequently and walk about. Truckers and others who must travel for long periods should try foam seat cushions to reduce road vibration. Arm rests are helpful in decreasing the force on the low back.

Back support. A simple back cushion can help greatly in any sitting situation where good back support is lacking.

Try a large folded towel or small blanket to find out what thickness works for you. When you have success, buy an inflatable pillow or commercial back support that can match the thickness you want.

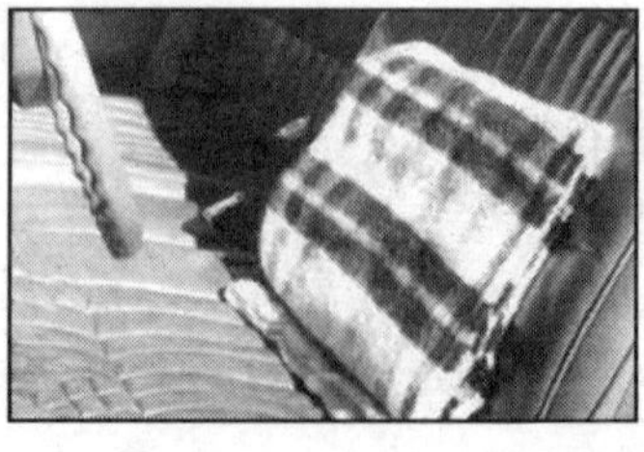

Lifting

Use these rules whenever you pick up anything. Use the basic ideas whenever you reach down or lean over, even if not exerting.

1. **Face the object.** Do not twist your body.
2. **Do the pelvic tilt.** Tuck in your buttocks and pull in your abdomen. Hold the tilt while you lift.
3. **Bend your knees.** Go down as far as possible with your legs, not your back.
4. **Hold object close** to your body. If the object can't be held close, don't lift it. Look straight ahead.
5. **Lift with your legs.** Use the large thigh muscles, not the small back muscles.
6. **Limit the height of your lift.** Lift a heavy load no higher than your waist. Lift a light load no higher than your shoulders. Greater height sways the back.
7. **Pivot on your feet.** When you must turn with an object in hand, turn your whole body. Do not twist to set the object down. *Twisting while bending is a major cause of injury.*

Combine these principles into one **habit of lifting.** It is not enough, for example, just to bend your knees. And don't be a hero with heavy items. If possible, get help with luggage. If an item is large or awkward to hold, at least two people should do the lifting.

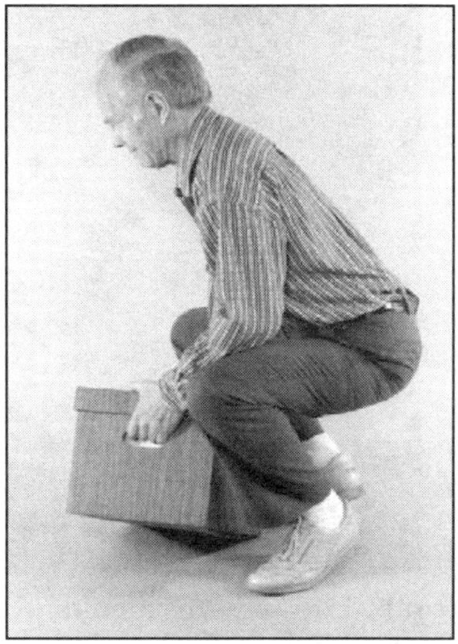

Pelvis tilted, knees bent

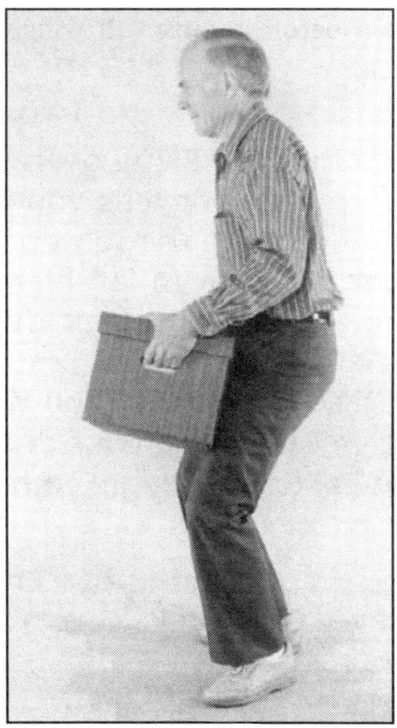

**Lift with legs.
Hold object close.**

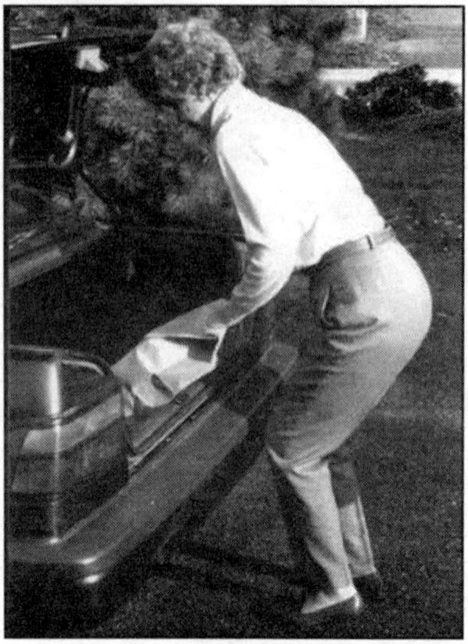

Crane Lift—use this method when you cannot use the squat lift (page 11). Bend knees slightly. Bend forward at hips, keeping head up and back straight. Slide object to you before taking full weight.

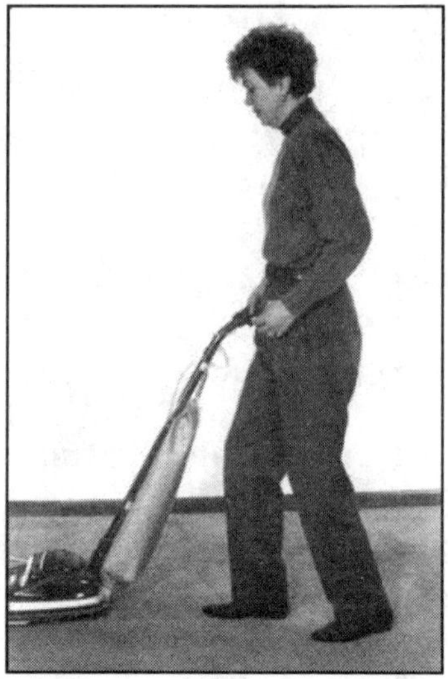

Bend knees when vacuuming, mopping, raking, etc. To avoid bending your back, step forward and backward as you work. If leaning is necessary, bend at your hips. Use self-propelled vacuum if possible.

Two Special Problems

Obesity. Being overweight puts an extra load on the spine. If your doctor tells you to lose weight, do the sensible things that will get the job done. Adopt a lifetime diet of smaller portions, low in fat, high in fruits and vegetables, with little or no alcohol, and very little refined sugar. Avoid diet fads. A regular exercise program of the type described on the next page is also important. You will burn more calories, even when not exercising. See your doctor before beginning any special diet or exercise program to be sure it is right for you. Remember, the more fat around your waist, the more strain on your back.

Sex. Back pain has a reputation for upsetting sexual relations. Severe pain calls for abstinence, but after pain has subsided, intercourse is usually okay. A suggestion: the person with the bad back should lie underneath and should use a pillow under the buttocks. An alternative is for the woman to lie on her side with knees bent. The man can lie behind, facing her back. A hot bath or gentle massage can be a helpful prelude.

FITNESS

Overall fitness requires exercise, proper weight, good diet, control of stress, and other healthy habits. Fitness has many rewards including a back less likely to cause pain.

Smoking can affect the back. A British study found that the more cigarettes a person smoked, the more severe and longer lasting were back attacks. Smoking reduces circulation in small blood vessels including those that nourish the spinal discs.

Good nutrition is important. Most people need to reduce fat intake and to increase vegetables, fruits, and whole grains. Supplements may be needed but will not make up for a poor diet. Extra **calcium** helps reduce age-related bone softening (osteoporosis). **Vitamin C** may be helpful because it helps build the collagen needed by discs. Some authorities believe 8 glasses of **water** a day will slow the disc-drying process.

Whole-body exercise is a part of fitness. *Aerobic exercise* is rhythmic motion done long enough and hard enough to keep your heart rate in the "target range" for at least 15 minutes. Longer periods, along with warm-up, are usually recommended. Exercising five or six days a week is best, but three days a week will probably maintain whatever level of fitness you achieve.

Be careful! Heavy exercise can be dangerous. An exercise program requires your doctor's approval and should always be increased in gradual stages. *It is not necessary to do any exercise at a strenuous level.* Some people should not try for the aerobic target but should just move at a comfortable pace.

The following activities are generally good, but heed the warnings that will be given.

- **Walking**
- **Bicycling**
- **Swimming**
- **Jogging**
- **Motorized Treadmill**
- **Certain other equipment**

Walking has low risk. It can also be done indoors, such as in a shopping mall, or on a motorized treadmill at home or in a gym. Work up to at least a half-hour per session. Some patients report back relief from walking one mile per day. *Important:* keep posture erect—no forward slumping. Let hips swing freely. Use well-cushioned shoes or special shock-absorbing insoles. Choose only level areas until your back is strong.

A motorized treadmill is the equipment people stick with most. Obviously, only what you continue to use will do you any good. A treadmill allows you to walk naturally at whatever pace you select. You can watch television or listen to music. Treadmills are expensive, but good used ones are available.

> *Caution:* Before you buy, be sure speed can be set low enough for your comfortable starting pace. Also look for a model with good shock absorption, especially if you intend to jog. Use *zero incline* until your back is strong. Some elderly people cannot get used to the "moving floor" and should consider a stationary bicycle.

Walking on a motorized treadmill is a good weight-bearing exercise.

Model with shock-absorbing belt is preferred.

Model must allow for adjustment to zero incline.

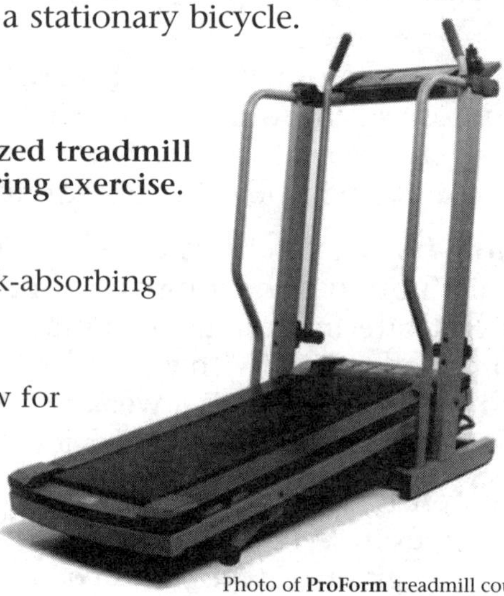

Photo of **ProForm** treadmill courtesy of Icon Health & Fitness, Inc., Logan, Utah.

Bicycling is best with minimum crouch and fully extended legs. The racing posture may strain the back unless the back is first strengthened and bike adjustments are ideal. Never ride with a swayed back. A **stationary exercise bicycle** is good for almost anyone (without arthritic knees) who has the will power to stay with it. Ride with a slightly rounded back.

Cross-country ski machines and **stair-steppers** may cause stress on the back because riders tend to lean forward.

A study found that exercise equipment injured over 25,000 people a year. Stationary bicycles were the most frequent cause, usually amputating a finger or toe. Children playing alone were the most frequent victims. Better, modern equipment has more safety features, but please take precautions.

Jog only with caution. *Avoid hard impact.* Reduce the shock with well-cushioned shoes and a running surface that gives. Look for a track with imitation grass or other cushioning material. Even so, jogging may not be right for you.

Swimming takes the load of gravity off the spine while allowing stretching, strengthening, and aerobic routines. If your doctor approves, learn an *endurance* program and use it on a regular basis. Avoid the butterfly and breast stroke at least until you are pain free. The side stroke is best for starting.

Conditional Activities. The following are hazardous for occasional players with backs out of condition. If you have strengthened your back with the back exercises, and if you play moderately and within your ability, your doctor might permit them. Most of these sports, however, are not effective exercise because exertion is intermittent (as in baseball) or just insufficient (bowling). Begin cautiously. If a certain movement causes back discomfort, either at the time or later, avoid that movement.

Baseball **Softball**	**Golf**—get coaching on how to protect the back. Do not lean backward after the swing.
Basketball	**Bowling**—do not jerk backward at release.
Table Tennis	**Tennis**—do not arch back as in hard service.
Horseback Riding	**Skiing**—hazardous for beginners. Experienced skiers must first get in shape.
Ice Skating	**Low-Impact Aerobic Exercise**—no jumping.
Back Packing	**Weight Lifting**—Get help from knowledgeable trainer. Avoid twisting, heavy weights, and bent-over positions, among others.

Hazardous Activities. Avoid these and *any others* that have rough contact, twisting, sudden impact, or direct stress on back.

Football	**Tobogganing**	**Certain Calisthenics:**
Touch Football	**Sledding**	**Both legs raised straight**
Soccer	**Snowmobiling**	**Sit-ups if legs straight**
Volleyball	**Ice Hockey**	**Hip twists, toe touches**
Handball	**Trampoline**	**Thrusting backward**

Nonetheless, if something in this hazardous category is important to you, perhaps you do not need to rule it out completely. After you are over your back pain and are in good shape, ask your doctor about it.

BACK EXERCISES

If you keep yourself fit through aerobic exercise and other good habits, you might not have to do back exercises. Yet even athletes with very good aerobic conditioning injure their backs. *With any history of back problems, back exercises are desirable and often necessary.* A daily 10 to 15 minute program will usually (1) eliminate pain and (2) protect against future attacks. You need to develop a program *individualized* for your needs. A physical therapist can help both in the selection of exercises and in making sure you are doing them correctly. If you do not have a physical therapist, use the following suggestions.

1. <u>WARM-UP.</u> **Begin with warm-up and relaxation activity.** Walking is good. See also "Relax Before Exercising," page 18.

2. <u>PAIN-RELIEF GROUP.</u> **Do one or more exercises from this group**, pages 5, 6, & 7. Those most often recommended are:
   - **Advanced Pelvic Tilt.** Page 7.
   - **Press-up** if backward bending helps you. Page 6.
   - **Double Knee to Chest** if forward bending helps. Page 7.

3. <u>CONDITIONING GROUP.</u> **Do at least three from this group.** The main purpose is to strengthen muscles around the spine.
   - **Partial Sit-up.** Helps almost everyone. Page 19.
   - **Diagonal Partial Sit-up.** Strengthens very important side and diagonal muscles missed by first sit-up. Page 19.
   - **Single Knee to Chest.** Almost always helps. Page 20.
   - **Half Knee Bend.** Strengthens the legs and thus helps with safer lifting and routine chores. Page 21.
   - **Wall Slide.** Another leg strengthening exercise. Page 21.
   - **Single Leg Raise.** Adds flexibility but is *not* for those in whom leg raises cause pain (sciatica). Page 22.
   - **Lying Back Arch.** Protects the back by strengthening muscles located *behind* the spine. Page 23.

Keep it simple—do exercises in the same order each day.

BE SURE TO READ THE "RULES," NEXT PAGE.

Rules for Back Exercises

1. **Start with physician's approval.** Do not begin the conditioning group if you still have acute (severe) pain.
2. **Exercise every day.** Benefits come from discipline.
3. **Do two sessions a day for two months.** By then you should see major improvement and can probably cut back to one session a day.
4. **Set aside regular, private times.** Usually these are an hour or so after arising and just before retiring. After arising, it's best to walk a few minutes first so that discs return to normal (they swell when not carrying weight).
5. **Select a comfortable, firm surface**—a carpeted or padded floor. Wear loose clothing or underclothes.
6. **Begin by relaxing.** See next page for a suggestion.
7. **Always move slowly and smoothly.** Do not jerk.
8. **Progress gradually at your own pace.** Do only *three repetitions* of each exercise you select in the conditioning group for the first two or three days. Then *add one repetition* to each exercise you can do with ease and comfort. When the new number can be done with ease and comfort, *add another.* Work up to 8 or 10. You can do more, but a short (10 to 15 minute) session is easier to stick with every day than a longer session.

Discomfort and soreness: At first, mild discomfort during exercise is common. So is stiffness or soreness between exercise periods. If this lasts beyond the first few days, you are probably exercising too hard or progressing too fast. Slow down. If it lasts more than the first two weeks, talk to your physician.

If you have significant discomfort or lingering pain or sensations from any exercise, stop that exercise for several days. Then try it again with fewer repetitions.

If leg pain is your main complaint (sciatica—see page 4), be sure to favor walking (page 13) and swimming (page 15). While you still have severe pain, however, avoid *any* activity or exercise which irritates your back. Hopefully, you will be helped by resting in a position of comfort (page 5) and by the other pain-relief positions and exercises, such as extension stretches (page 6) and perhaps the pelvic tilt (page 7). As pain subsides, continue pain-relief positions and move slowly into the conditioning group (page 19 and following). You will not be able to do the *single-leg raise* while this condition persists.

Relax Before Each Exercise Session

Heat helps. You may have found already that heat on your low back (tub bath, shower, heating pad) for 15 to 20 minutes relieves discomfort. Much of the benefit is because heat relaxes muscles. So, even if you have no pain at the time, using heat before exercise will help with relaxation.

A relaxation exercise helps. The following is one of many possibilities. Do this or a substitute before each exercise session.

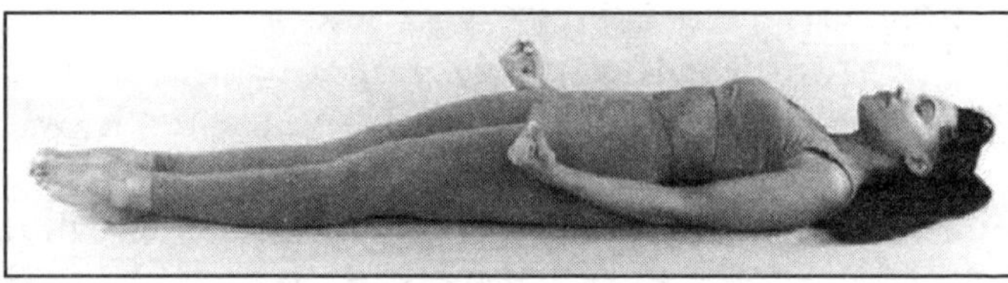

Body Tightener/Relaxer

1. **Lie on your back on covered floor.**
2. **Tighten your whole body as you take a slow, deep breath. Clench fists and press legs together.**
3. **Close your eyes and "let go" of your body as you exhale. Let arms and legs "drift away," Let your jaw sag.**

Repeat 5 times.

To make sure you follow the instruction, have someone else read the instruction while you do the exercise.

PARTIAL SIT-UP

Strengthens low back and abdominal muscles

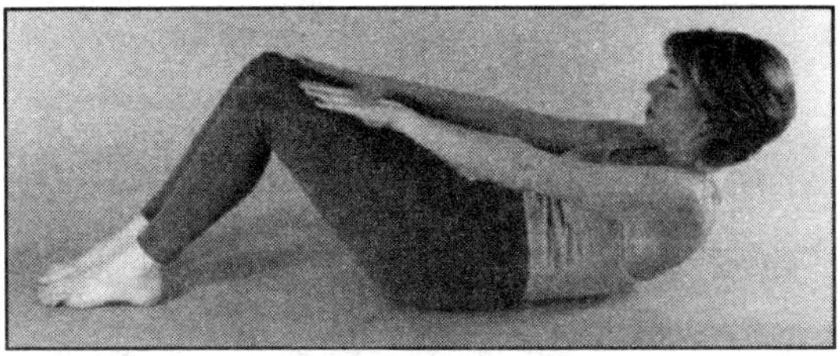

1. **Start on your back, knees bent. Do the pelvic tilt and hold back flat on floor as you begin next step.**
2. **Extend hands toward knees. Slowly raise head and neck, then shoulders. Use a curl-up motion, keeping chin toward chest. Hold for a count of 5.**
3. **Curl down to starting position. Relax and repeat for a total of 3 times. Gradually increase to 8 or 10 times.**

Benefit begins when shoulder blades leave floor, but at first you might not be able to raise them very far. That's okay. *Gradually* go higher until back is 45 to 60 degrees from floor. This may take weeks, or you may never get that high. That's okay too. Also, a full sit-up is unnecessary and may irritate the low back.

ADVANCED SIT-UPS. Some lightweights may find the above easy. They can advance with arms at waist, then with hands at ears. Do not lock hands behind head (creates pull on head).

DIAGONAL PARTIAL SIT-UP

Strengthens side and diagonal abdominal muscles

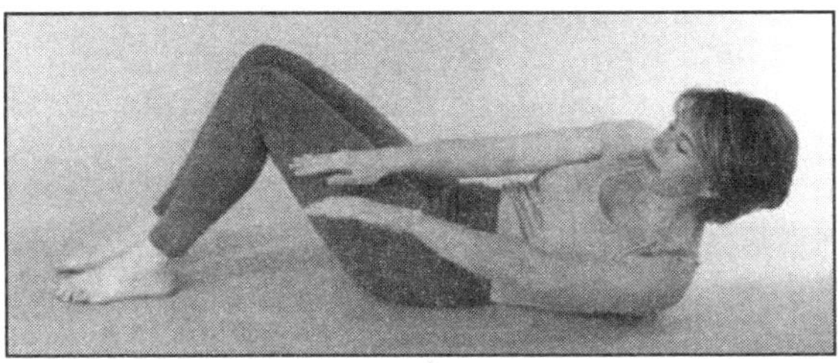

1. **Start as above. Do pelvic tilt and hold back flat on floor.**
2. **Curl as above, but reach with both hands to side of knees, gently turning trunk and shoulders. Hold for 5 count.**
3. **Curl back, relax, repeat but reach to other side of knees. Do 3 times to each side. Work up to 8 or 10.**

Caution: Never do sit-ups with legs straight! Never jerk for height!

SINGLE KNEE TO CHEST

Stretches low back and hamstrings.
Stretches hip flexors (when legs extended).

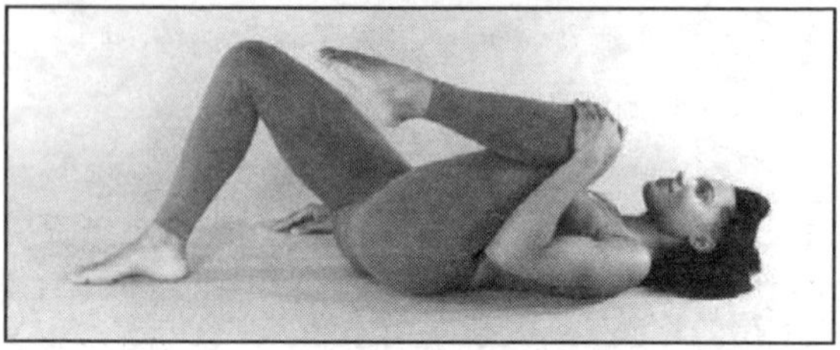

START on back on covered floor, knees bent.

1. Do the pelvic tilt so that your low back is flat on floor.
2. With hand over (or under) one knee, pull knee gently toward armpit. When you feel tension, stop (gradually you will go farther). Hold for a slow count of 5.
3. Return to starting position. Relax a few seconds.
4. Repeat with the other knee, starting with back flat. Do each knee 3 times. Gradually increase to 8 or 10.

Advanced exercise

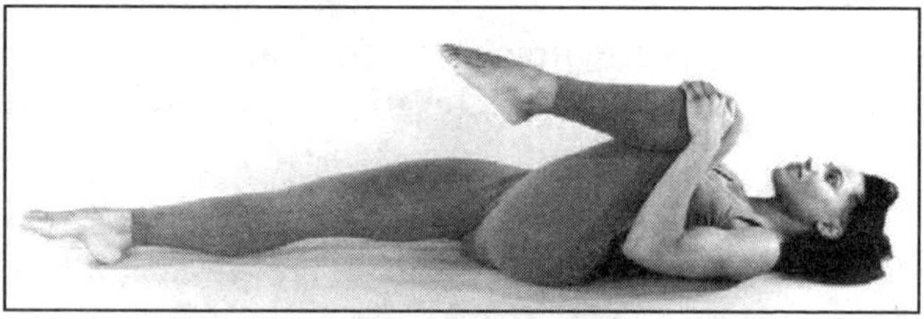

After a few weeks, when you can more easily keep the low back flat on the floor, start with both legs straight. First do the pelvic tilt, then bend one knee, then pull it over chest. Hold for a count of 5. Keep the opposite leg straight and on the floor so as to stretch the hip-flexing muscles attached to that leg. Return the pulled knee to the bent resting position. Slide foot so that both legs are straight on floor again. Repeat with other knee. Increase number of repetitions gradually.

The pelvic tilt is an important part of this exercise and others. Do not allow the back to arch.

HALF KNEE BEND

Strengthens hamstrings and quadriceps. Prepares for lifting and other tasks using leg muscles, not back.

Caution: Discontinue this exercise if it causes significant and persisting discomfort in knees or hips.

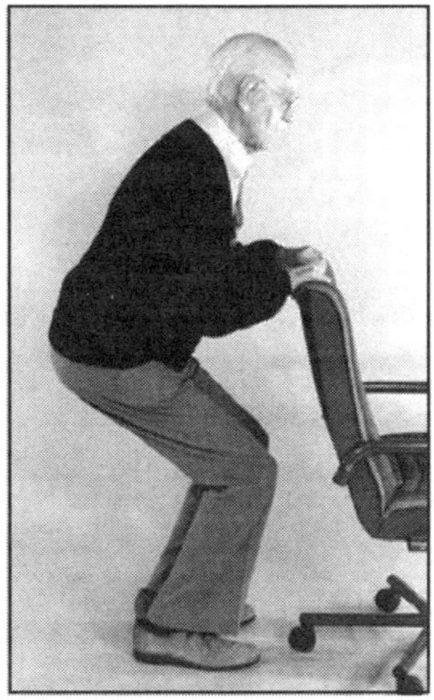

Begin after 3 or 4 weeks, when you can do a good pelvic tilt. Have someone confirm that you are holding a flat back during the exercise.

START by standing behind a sofa, heavy chair, or next to a counter, holding it for balance.

1. **Do the pelvic tilt and hold it.**
2. **Squat down ABOUT HALF WAY, only as far as is comfortable.**
3. **Stand up, using leg power, not hands. Do not bounce.**

Relax and repeat twice, increasing gradually to 8 to 10 times.

WALL SLIDE

This alternative to above exercise may be easier than the above if you stop the slide at about 45 degrees.

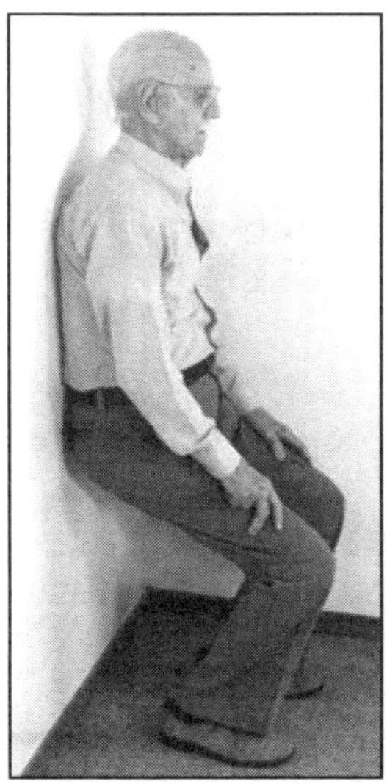

START by standing with back against a smooth wall. Place heels about 12 inches from wall.

1. **Do the pelvic tilt so that back is flat against wall.**
2. **Slowly slide back down wall until thighs are at about 45 degrees. Hold for a few seconds, gradually increasing to a count of 10 or more.**
3. **Slide up, relax, and repeat.**

ADVANCED EXERCISE: Slide to 90 degrees as if sitting in a chair. If you can, gradually work up to a hold of 30 seconds or more.

SINGLE-LEG RAISE

Stretches low back and hamstrings. Strengthens abdominal and hip-flexing muscles. Stretches hip-flexing muscles (when both legs extended).

If you have sciatica (dominant leg pain), omit this exercise.

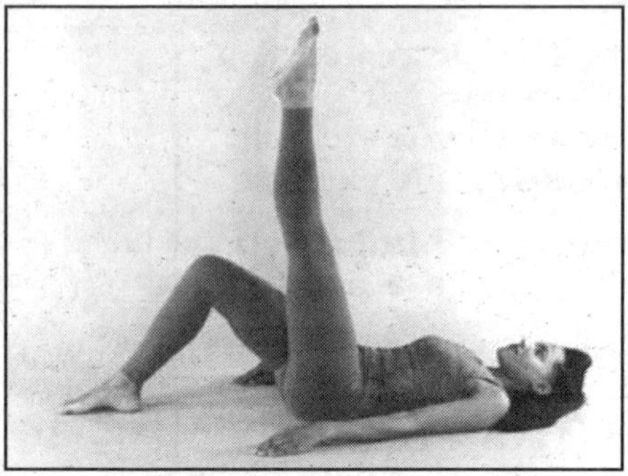

START on your back on covered floor, ONE knee bent.

1. **Do the pelvic tilt so that you begin with back flat on floor.**
2. **Slowly raise straight leg, keeping it straight and keeping low back on floor. Raise leg *until you feel mild tension. Do not thrust.* Greater height comes gradually. Hold for a slow count of 5.**
3. **Slowly lower leg, flattening back as leg approaches floor.**
4. **Relax a few seconds and repeat with other leg. Raise each leg a total of 3 times, increasing gradually to 8 or 10.**

Advanced exercise

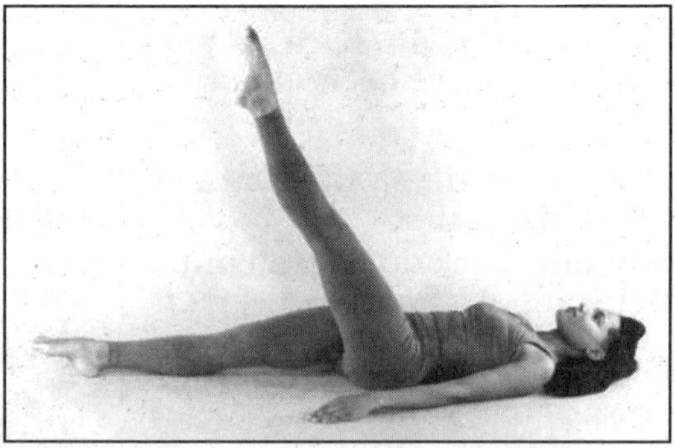

After 4 to 6 weeks, you can probably do the pelvic tilt with legs straight without discomfort. If so, try starting the above exercise with both legs straight. The low back now tends to rise. Check with your hand to be sure that it does not—both when lifting the leg and lowering it. If you cannot hold your low back against the floor, resume with one knee bent.

LYING BACK ARCH (extension)

Strengthens erector spinae group running length of spine. Improves posture.

Advance after you can do the previous level well 8 to 10 times. DO NOT JERK upward. Do not continue at any level that causes pain.

Level 1

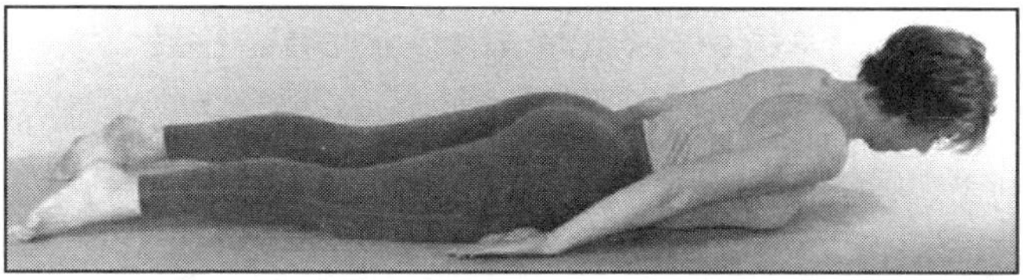

START: Face down on floor, chin tucked in, arms at sides.

1. Slowly raise head and chest as much as you can. Keep head down, chin tucked in. Hold for slow 5 count. Breath normally.
2. Slowly return to floor.
3. Relax. Repeat twice. Gradually increase to 8 or 10.

Level 2

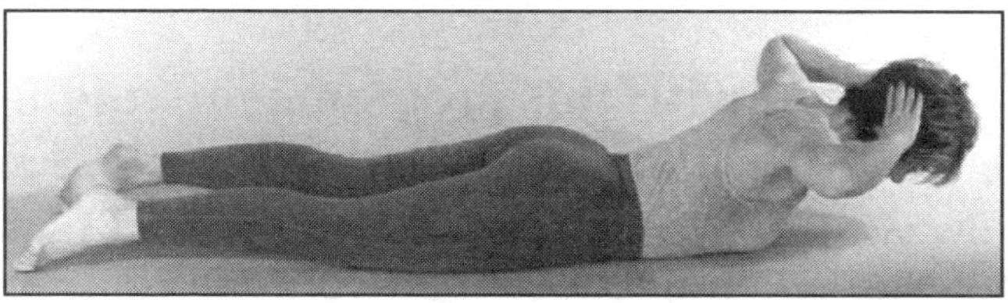

Same as Level 1 except hold hands at head, elbows off floor.

Level 3
Advanced

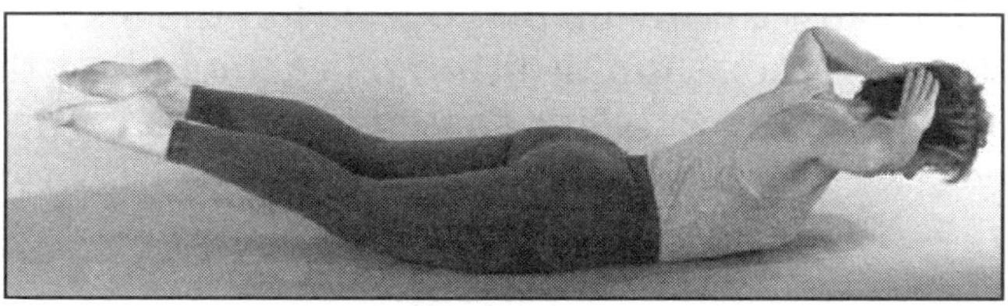

Same as Level 2 except raise legs (keep straight) *and* upper body.

Level 4
Very advanced

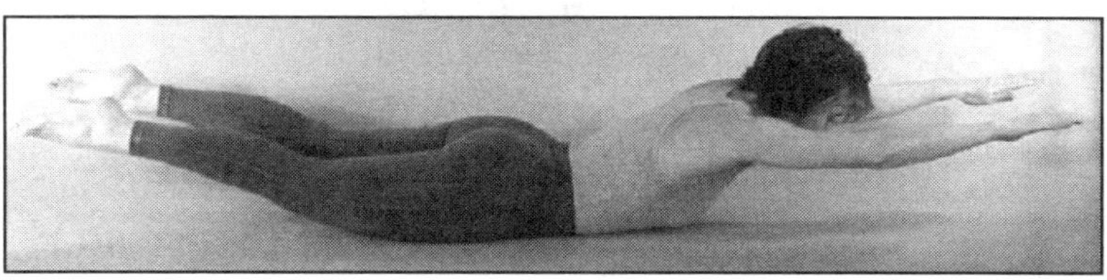

Same as Level 3 except raise outstretched arms also.

Level 5—*Advanced Endurance.* Offers greatest benefit, but takes more time. Leave arms at sides. Raise upper body and legs (keep straight). Hold the position until you tire. Gradually work toward 4 minutes.

Exercises are important, but . . .

Exercises are not a *total* control program for back problems. They improve strength, flexibility, circulation, alignment, and posture, and that makes exercise important. But so are all the other subjects discussed in this booklet. Daily habits and activities need to be protective. That means, for example, lifting and doing other chores the safe way. It means developing habits that lead to overall physical fitness. These things are all in your hands.

Even with this program, you might have another back attack, but. . . .

Now you know what to do. Be quick about it. Rush to the pain-relief measures that work for you. Take the load off your spine, such as with the "Z" position, page 5, or by just curling up on your side in the fetal position. Other positions might bring relief, including the Half Knee Bend or Wall Slide shown on page 21. *The quicker you "unload" your spine, the more likely you will avoid painful muscle spasm.*

Plan on a return to normal life.

Don't suddenly begin anything vigorous, but gradually work into normal activities. Don't walk about as if you were on egg shells. Worrying causes tension, and tension is not good for the spine. Instead, expect progress. Keep in touch with your doctor, and be sure to see him or her if there is no progress. But that's unlikely. Nearly everyone gets better on this program.